THE KETOGENIC DIET

Benefit or harm? Rules. Menu.

Stella Parker

Table of Contents

The origin

Originally used for children with epilepsy to reduce seizures, the ketogenic diet was developed in the 1920s after demonstrating anticonvulsant effects in epilepsy. The regime, however, has gained popularity in recent years as a quick way to lose weight but also for improving the symptoms of type 2 diabetes and cardiovascular disease. This diet is now experiencing a renewed interest from doctors and researchers because of its therapeutic potential.

What is the ketogenic diet?

The ketogenic diet is an isocaloric diet that is rich in fat (about 80% of the calories consumed each day are derived from lipids) and very low in carbohydrates (20 to 40 g per day depending on the tolerance level of each), which allows the body to modify its metabolism without being hungry. This regime is distinguished by the appearance of bodies called "ketones" in blood and urine. The liver produces ketones from fat whenever the body has fasted for more than one day or has absorbed sufficient calories from fat without being accompanied by added fat. Among the ketones are acetoacetic acid, acetone (which is removed by exhaling and produces a "fruity" smell when a person is suddenly in strong ketosis), and beta-hydroxybutyric acid. Chemically speaking, the latter is not a ketone, but physiologically, it is assimilated to ketones because it appears wherever there is a production of acetoacetic acid.

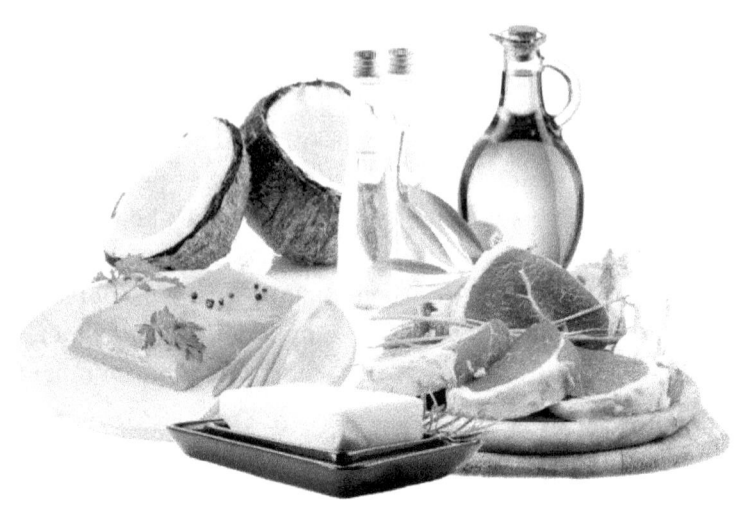

Permitted and avoidable foods:

Food allowed:

Fish, seafood, meat, poultry, eggs, butter, vegetable oil, vinegar, juice of lemon, olives, avocado, low-carbohydrate vegetables such as leafy green vegetables (spinach, lettuce of all types, endive, cabbage kale, chard), and cheese farms (maximum 100 g per day).

Foods allowed in moderation:

Dairy products such as milk (preferred whole milk 3.25%), Mediterranean yogurts likely to be 7-8% fat, more vegetables rich in carbohydrates (avoid carrots, beets, corn, parsnips, apple Earth, sweet potato, spaghetti squash, and green peas), wine, strong alcohol, and coffee without sugar.

Foods to avoid:

- sugar,
- sugary products,
- grain products (breakfast cereals, bread, pasta, rice, couscous, quinoa, oatmeal, barley, buckwheat, crackers, muffins, pancakes, tortillas, pita, bagels, granola bar, and any other product made from flour such as pastries, donuts, biscuits, sweets),
- legumes,
- fruit (except berries which in some cases are allowed), soft cheeses (cottage, ricotta),
- Fresh cheese,
- rice-based and soy-based cheeses

- soft drinks, frozen desserts (frozen cream and yogurt), chocolate, white sugar, brown sugar, honey, maple syrup, Molasses, jams, fruit and vegetable juices, cereal, coffees, sweet sauces, flavored soy milk or beverages, fruit compotes and fruit salads with added sugar.

Taking a multivitamin and a fiber supplement is recommended. Besides, it is recommended to stay well hydrated by drinking 2.5 to 3 liters of water per day.

Types of fat to be preferred

As a significant amount of fat is ingested every day, it is important to care about the kind of fat. It is recommended to limit consumption of omega-6 fatty acid, which in excess, has a pro-inflammatory effect. The primary sources of omega-6 are soybean oils, corn, safflower, grapeseed, sunflower, and wheat germ. It is, therefore, necessary to limit the consumption of salad dressings, vinaigrettes, and mayonnaises based on these oils.

The consumption of monounsaturated fats (olive oil, avocado, and nuts) and saturated fats (cuts of fatty meat, and dairy products rich in fat) is advisable. The use of coconut oil is also recommended because it contains fat that is quickly processed into ketones.

Ketogenic diet for weight loss

According to various studies, the ketogenic diet for weight loss is characterized by the maximum consumption of 50 g of carbs per day, representing around 5% of the calories consumed in the day. A typical diet usually provides between 45 and 65% of our calories in the form of carbohydrates. The remainder is distributed between lipids and proteins. In the ketogenic diet, the calories ingested in the form of lipids can reach up to 75%, and the proteins occupy the remaining 20%.

How does the ketogenic diet necessitate weight loss?

Usually, the body draws in the carbohydrates consumed in the day to the energy needed for proper functioning of the body. In this diet, with carbohydrates being extremely limited, the body begins to tap into the carbohydrates that are stored in the muscles and liver called "glycogen" stores. As each gram of glycogen is bound to 3-4 g of water in the body, significant early weight loss in the ketogenic diet is actually a loss of water. When glycogen stores are depleted, the body begins to use lipids or fats to produce energy. When the body uses fat in the absence of carbohydrates, it produces waste products called ketones. Next, the ketone bodies begin to accumulate in the blood and their odor, similar to that of nail polish, becomes perceptible in the breath. This is the primary indicator that the body is in a "ketosis" state. It takes around 2 to 4 weeks before arriving at this condition. The state of "ketosis" can be checked by obtaining strips of a urine analysis in the pharmacy.

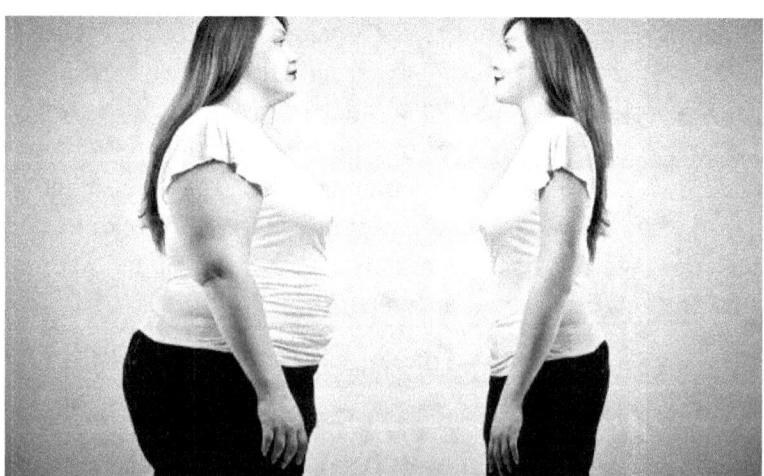

This state of "ketosis" causes a marked decrease in appetite, which contributes to reducing the amount of food consumed. This condition can also lead to nausea and fatigue. Although the scheme does not center on counting calories, those who follow the diet absorb fewer calories because they do not go hungry, and this, therefore, leads to weight loss.

Tips to lose weight with the ketogenic diet

- You have to have a composition table of food and a culinary balance available to quantify carbohydrates accurately.
- When tired, do not hesitate to take a vitamin supplementation.
- It is imperative to raise revenues ahead of plan. Cooking with the energy distribution imposed by the diet will otherwise quickly become a real headache.

In total, if the ketogenic diet can give a boost to losing 2 or 3 pounds quickly on a particular occasion, it cannot be followed long-term without health risks.

Example of a ketogenic menu providing 1500 kcal

Breakfast

- Unsweetened coffee or tea (possibility of sweetener)
- 1 handful (30 g) of almonds, walnuts or hazelnuts
- 50 g of red fruits: strawberries, raspberries, blackcurrants, gooseberries

Lunch and dinner

- 50 g of raw vegetables (the equivalent of a small grated carrot), vinaigrette with 1 tablespoon of walnut or rapeseed oil
- 120 g of meat or fish or 2 eggs: cooking with 1 tablespoon of colza or olive oil
- 100 g vegetables + 2 teaspoons of butter or 2 tablespoons of whole cream
- To taste
- 60 g of cheese or 30 g of cheese + 1 ramekin of whole milk white cheese

Why is the ketogenic diet used for epilepsy?

When sugar is not supplied to the body, it is the ketones that provide the brain with the energy it needs. Cerebral cells are very fond of these ketones, which are particularly effective - this is perhaps why the ketogenic diet is often highly effective for epileptics, whose seizures decrease or even disappear completely. Muscles and organs can draw their energy directly into fatty acids from either body fat stores or fat-rich foods such as butter, nuts, oils and the like. They do not need ketones. In theory, a large part of the brain cells could also function by exploiting the fatty acids. However, inside the cells, fatty acids burn with relatively low efficiency: they require a lot of oxygen, produce large amounts of "free radicals" and related reactive species to oxygen (ERO) harmful to cells, and their energy production is relatively slow. These three factors render them incapable of supplying sufficient energy to the brain, an extremely active and sensitive organ. This is why the mitochondria of nerve cells of the brain are not designed for this inefficient and harmful form of fat burning, and the key enzymes necessary for the degradation of fatty acids (beta-oxidation) are only present in very small quantities. On the other hand, the combustion of ketones in the mitochondria is extremely effective in comparison to that of glucose and its rapid and very clean because it produces little ERO. This process can be compared to the operation of a car engine. The simplest motors work perfectly with regular gasoline. Cars equipped with a powerful engine demand Super, and Formula 1 cars even work with superior quality fuel, a kind of "super super" - they would go on in slow motion if they were driven with Regular gasoline. As "Formula 1 cells" in our body, cells in our brain cannot function by burning amino acids (which is equivalent to ordinary gasoline): they need at least super (glucose) or, even better, gasoline for Formula 1 (ketones).

How can people with cancer benefit from this regime?

Fatty acids are the ideal energy provider for all the cells of our body except those of the brain. Cancer patients need particularly high amounts of fat to maintain muscle mass and maintain sufficient physical strength. Indeed, cancer modifies the metabolism in such a way that the muscles react less well to the signal of insulin. Like people with diabetes, cancer patients become insulin-resistant, which has the effect of lessening the capacity of their muscles to exploit sugar as a source of energy. When their cells lack sugar and do not have sufficient fatty acids to compensate, people become weak and quickly deplete. Unfortunately, many cancer patients are unaware of this situation. Unlike sugar, fatty acids can penetrate cells without being dependent on insulin. And when enough fat is put at the disposal of an organism, as is the case with a diet low in carbohydrates and high in fat, or a ketogenic diet, the muscles regain energy including in cases of proven insulin resistance. All the endurance sportsmen know this phenomenon: it is the mode "burning of fat" that makes it possible to run a marathon without being obliged to continuously absorb foods rich in sugar.

Principle of the ketogenic diet: to mimic the effects of fasting

This diet, which is part of the low-carbohydrate diets, aims to reduce the blood sugar levels, forcing the body to adapt (glucose is the primary fuel of the body):

The body then produces its energy through its fat reserves that turn into ketone bodies.

The difference with the fasting is that the ketogenic diet fat intake is increased to encourage ketosis and not to cause muscle wasting. The body draws its energy in the carbohydrates, then in the lipids, and finally, in the proteins.

KETOGENIC RECIPES

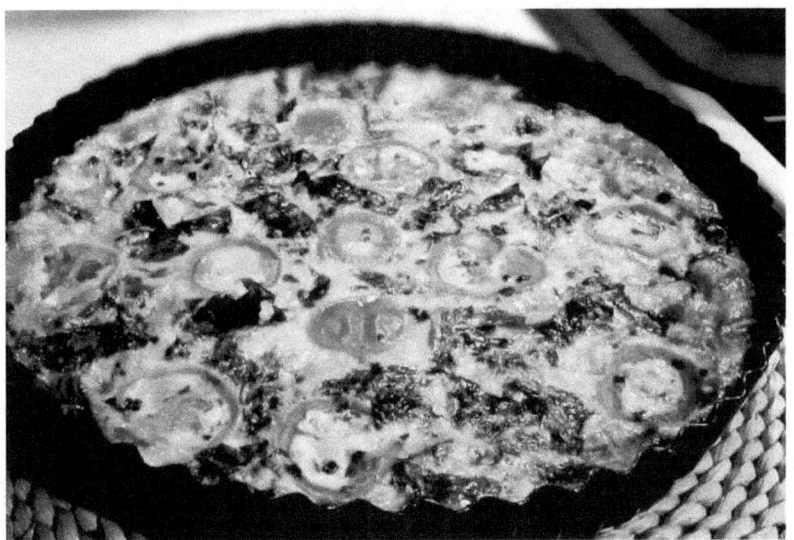

Flourless quiche

Prep time 5mins. Cooking time 20mins. 8 servings.

Ingredients
- 12 eggs
- 5 cl fresh cream
- 100g grated cheese
- A clove of garlic
- 100g mushrooms in 2 tablespoons of olive oil
- 10 cherry tomatoes, halved
- 50g of pitted green olives, sliced

Preparation
- In a bowl, beat the eggs, add all ingredients, mix well and put in a quiche dish. Bake for 15 minutes at 180 degrees.

- Careful preparation can swell in the oven and overflow from the mold if it is too low.

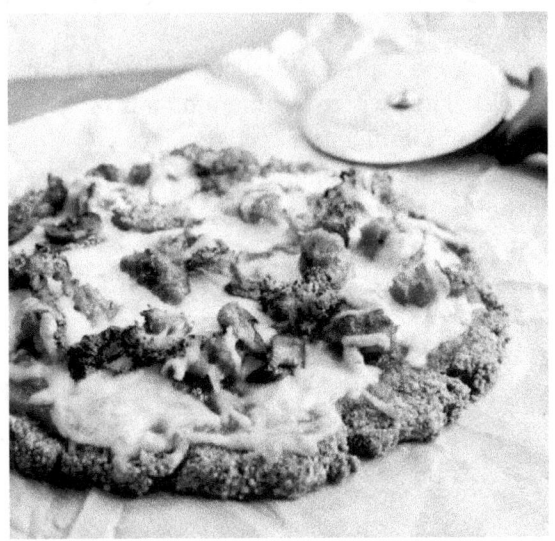

Flax seeds and cheese pizza

Prep time 5mins. Cooking time 20mins. 1 pizza.

Ingredients
- For the pizza base:
- 200g grated mozzarella for dough
- 4 tablespoons grated Parmesan cheese
- 50g ground flaxseed
- ½ glass of water
- A clove of garlic grated
- Salt and pepper
- 1 egg

For the filling:
- 6 tablespoons tomato sauce
- Topping of choice (pepperoni, hamburger, tuna, etc.)
- 100g grated cheese

Preparation

- In a bowl, mix all ingredients for the dough vigorously to avoid any lumps.
- Create a round-shaped spread 25-30cm in diameter on a baking oven dish, lined with parchment paper.
- Bake at 150 degrees until batter is golden.
- Garnish like a pizza and put on the grill.
- Cool slightly before serving.

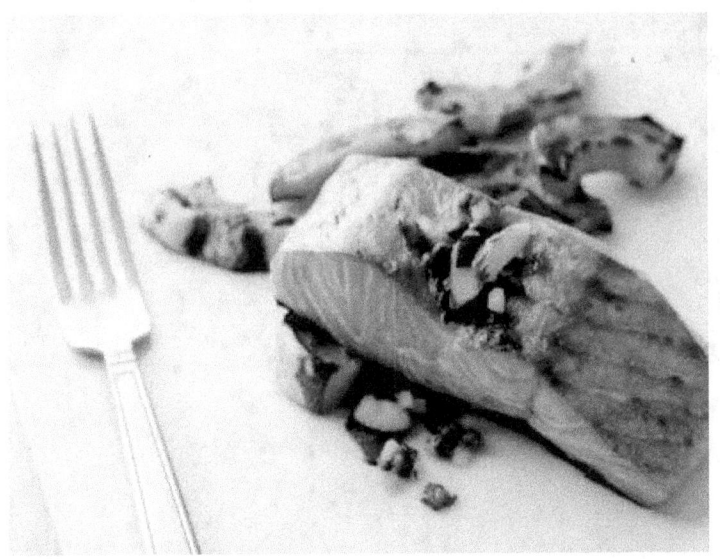

Baked Salmon

Prep time 8mins. Cooking time 25mins. 3 servings.

Ingredients
- A beautiful salmon fillet 400g
- 2 tablespoons mustard
- 2 tablespoons olive oil
- Juice of half a lemon
- 4 tablespoons chopped chives
- Salt and pepper

Preparation
- Combine mustard, olive oil, lemon juice, 3 tablespoons of chives cut, salt and pepper. Coat the salmon steak with this mixture and place on a baking dish.
- Bake for 15-20 minutes at 180°. We need the salmon to remain soft. Serve with blanched vegetables in olive oil, garlic, and parsley.

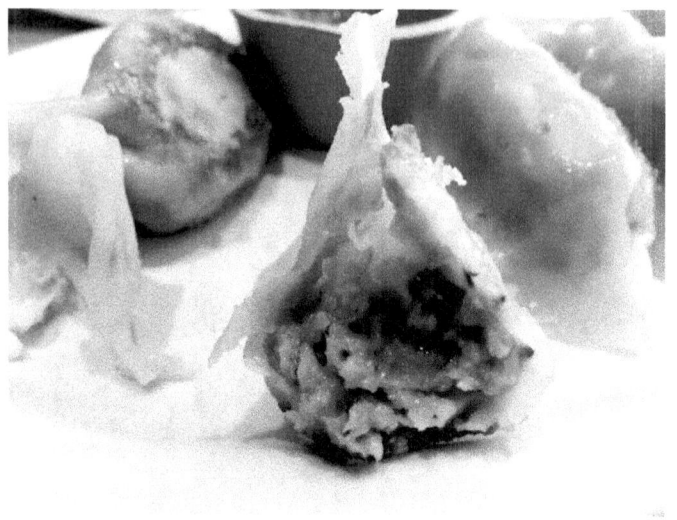

Chicken dumplings filled with cheese

Prep time 5mins. Cooking time 20mins. 3 servings.

Ingredients
- 300g turkey or ground chicken
- Emmental cheese, diced
- Salt
- Pepper
- Nutmeg
- ½ grated onion (2 tablespoons)
- 1 clove garlic, minced

Preparation
- Mix ground chicken with spices and onion and chopped garlic, make dumplings with the Emmental center cubes. Put in an oiled dish in the oven.
- Cook until the dumplings are golden.

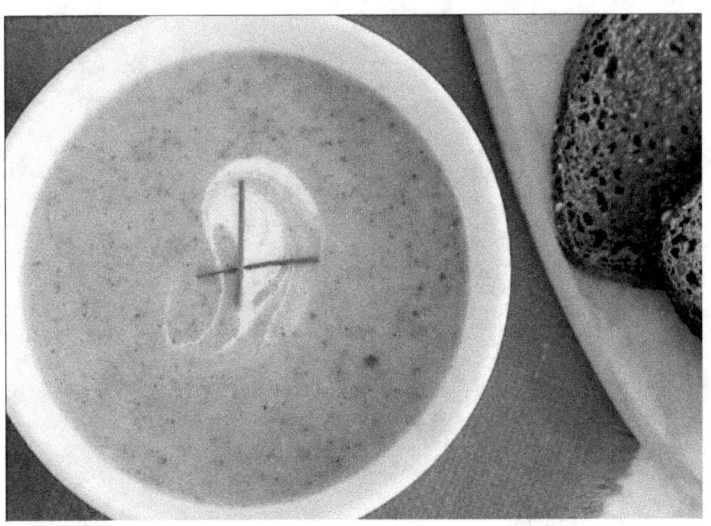

Broccoli and zucchini soup

Prep time 6mins. Cooking time 22mins. 5 servings.

Ingredients
- 400g broccoli, washed and chopped
- 200g of zucchini, diced
- 1 leek
- 50g butter
- Salt and pepper
- Cheese

Preparation:
- In a pan, melt the butter. Add the leek cut and melt. Then add the chopped vegetables, mixing well.
- Wet vegetables, cover and cook for twenty minutes. Vegetables should be melting.
- Mix everything with cheese to make a soup, add salt and pepper to taste and enjoy!

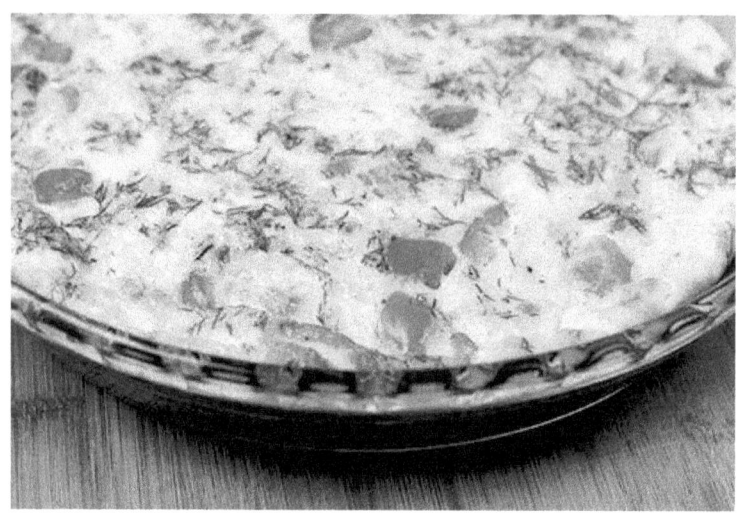

Quiche without crust

Prep time 5mins. Cooking time 20mins. 3 portions.

Ingredients
- 8 eggs
- 1 bowl of fresh cream
- 1 bowl of grated cheese
- Salt and pepper
- 1 clove of garlic, minced
- Filling: 100g fried mushrooms, 100 or 100g of shrimp cooked, ground meat and 100g of peppers, or cooked chicken breast and 100g feta

Preparation
- Beat eggs with cream, chopped clove of garlic, and salt and pepper in a bowl.
- Place the toppings of your choice into muffin molds and pour over eggs.
- Bake at 180 degrees for 15 minutes.

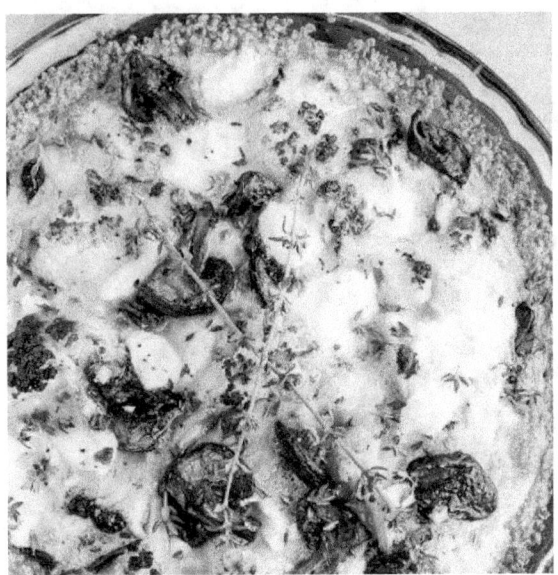

Mini quiches cauliflower and mushrooms

Prep time 5mins. Cooking time 20mins. 8 portions.

Ingredients
- A cauliflower half-head
- 200g of Paris mushrooms
- 6 eggs
- 5 cl fresh cream
- A clove of minced garlic
- 2 tablespoons of chopped chives
- 50g butter
- 100g grated cheese
- Salt and pepper

Preparation
- Cook the cauliflower steamed, cool, and mash with a fork.
- Fry the sliced mushrooms in butter. Mix with remaining ingredients and place in muffin tins.

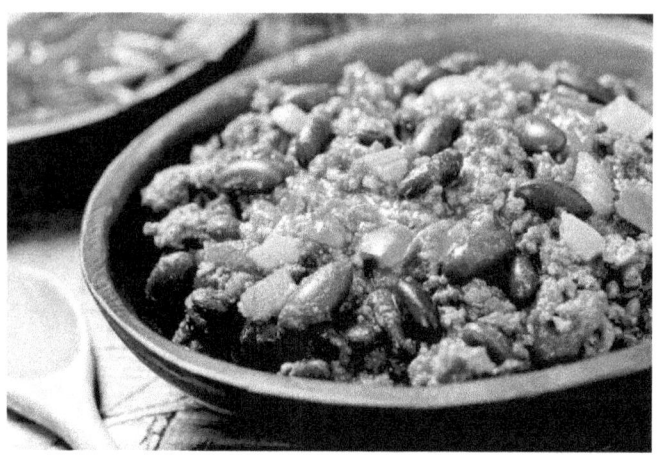

Chili con carne

Prep time 5mins. Cooking time 1h 10mins. 6 servings.

Ingredients
- 750g of minced meat with fat
- 1 medium onion
- 3 green peppers
- 3 tablespoons tomato paste
- 1 tomato, diced
- 1 tablespoon Mexican seasoning
- 2 garlic cloves
- 5 cl olive oil
- Salt and pepper

Preparation
- Cut the onion and diced peppers, crush the garlic and fry in a pan with half of the olive oil
- Fry the minced meat, add salt and pepper.
- Add the chopped tomatoes and diced tomato paste to the pot with the Mexican seasoning, then add the rest of the olive oil and cooked ground meat.
- Cook everything over a very low heat for one hour.

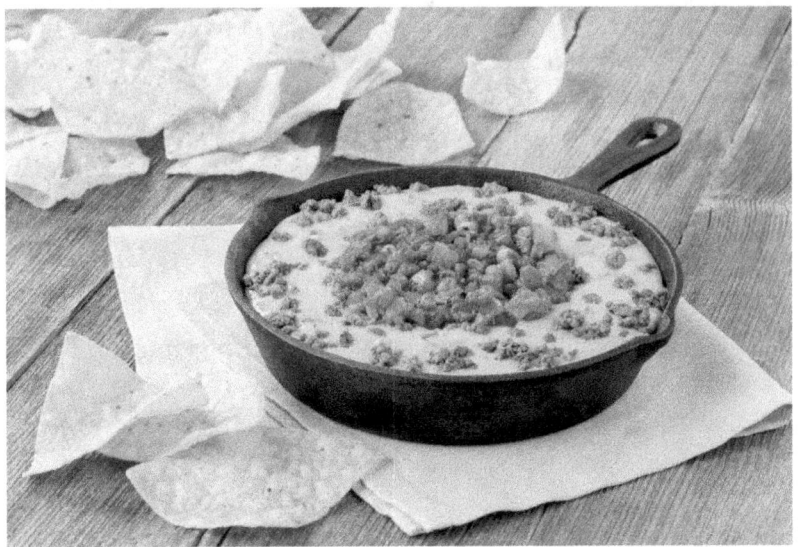

Queso fundido meat

Prep time 5mins. Cooking time 30mins. 6 servings.

Ingredients
- 200g of minced meat
- A small onion knife
- 1 bowl of green, yellow and red peppers, diced
- 200g of grated mozzarella
- 200g of grated Cheddar or Edam
- A pinch of pepper
- 1 tomato, diced
- 3 tablespoons of chopped cilantro
- 2 tablespoon of olive oil
- 1 clove garlic, chopped

Preparation
- Preheat oven to 200°. fry salted minced meat and pepper in a pan with a tablespoon of olive oil. Remove from heat and reserve the meat.

- In the same skillet, pour a tablespoon of olive oil, a clove of minced garlic, onion, and peppers, cook until the onion becomes translucent. There should not be any liquid in the pan.
- In a baking dish (a cast iron skillet, or fried for paella), place a layer of meat, vegetables and cheese mixture. The final layer will be of cheese and sprinkle with pepper.
- Bake for 10 minutes. We need the cheese to melt completely but do not let it harden. After taking out of the over, decorate the dish with crushed tomatoes and chopped coriander.
- Serve

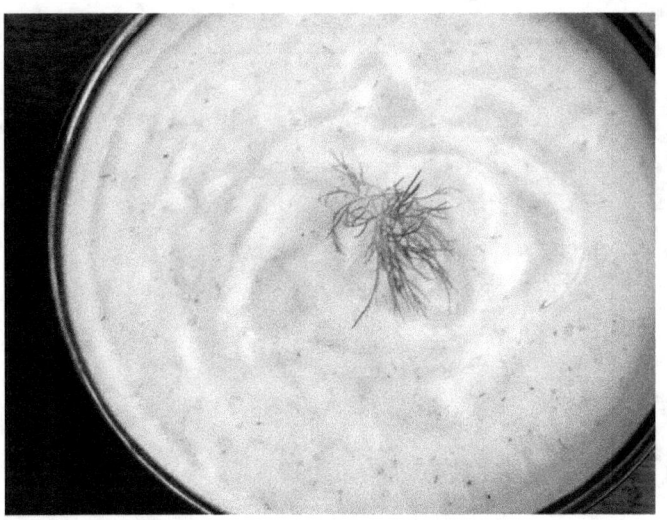

Cauliflower cream

Prep time 8mins. Cooking time 25mins. 3 servings.

Ingredients
- 1 medium cauliflower
- 1 half onion
- Half a box of Philadelphia or Jebly herb
- 50g butter
- Salt and pepper
- 1 liter of chicken stock

Preparation
- Put the butter melt in a pan, add half an onion and cauliflower cut pieces. Add salt and pepper, cover with broth.
- Cook for 20 minutes from the rotation of the valve.
- Mix everything with Philadelphia cheese with herbs.

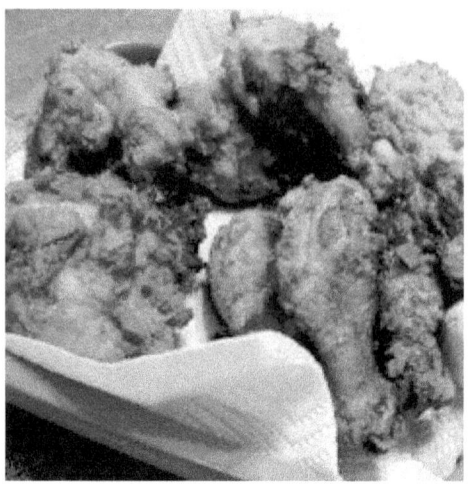

Fried chicken with coconut flour

Prep time 5mins. Cooking time 20mins. 6 servings.

Ingredients
- 2kg of chicken thighs (up and pestle)
- Salt and pepper
- Garlic powder or two garlic cloves mashed
- 1 tablespoon paprika
- 100g of coconut flour
- Oil for frying

Preparation
- Marinade: In a large bowl, combine the chicken, salt, pepper, garlic, and paprika. Mix well with your hands and make sure the spices cover the entire surface of the chicken. Marinade for at least two hours. It is better to marinade the night before.
- Breading the chicken marinated in coconut flour, heat oil in a deep fryer or saucepan to 190°. Fry the chicken being careful not to put too much at once so that the chicken becomes crispy. Cook for 8 minutes on each side until the chicken pieces are golden.

- Cut the chicken in two to make sure the meat is not pink in the interior.

Advantages and disadvantages of the ketogenic diet

Advantages

- The ketogenic diet gives you the opportunity to eat fatty meats or cheeses, which are considered better gustative products since fats convey aromas.
- The fatty substances present in large quantities make the dishes attractive and not too dry as is the case in most diets. It also allows for a variation of preparation: gratins, sauces, fries, etc.
- From a nutritional standpoint, the ketogenic diet largely covers the needs of Omega 3 and vitamin E. These essential fats are missing in most dishes.
- The fat allows a fast satiety, so it is quite easy to respect the quantities proposed.

Disadvantages

- In the short-term, the removal (or so) of carbohydrates can cause hypoglycemia, causing tiredness and headaches. The initiation of the ketosis process is frequently accompanied by nausea and induces bad breath (due to acetone released by the lungs) that tends to persist.
- The ketogenic diet can cause digestive problems: sometimes diarrhea, but more often constipation, given its limited fiber intake (not starchy, some vegetables and fruits).
- In the long-term, the ketogenic diet may promote cardiovascular disease. First, because the diets providing

over 40% of energy intake as fat induce atherosclerosis (clogged arteries), the other for a lack of protective nutrients such as fiber, vitamins (C and beta-carotene), and polyphenols in fruits and vegetables. A complementation is not necessarily effective since there are 2,000 different polyphenols distributed in the plants.

- It is a diet that excludes many foods such as bread and starches, sugar products and some fruits; it seems difficult to hold long-term and can probably cause eating disorders.

The trademarks that are used are without any consent, and the publication of the trademark is without permission or backing by the trademark owner. All trademarks and brands within this book are for clarifying purposes only and are the owned by the owners themselves, not affiliated with this document.

www.ingramcontent.com/pod-product-compliance
Lightning Source LLC
Chambersburg PA
CBHW071322280526
45788CB00004B/1983